Sleeping Clean

The New Trend in Healthcare

Improve Your Health With More Restful Sleep

RON KNESS

Contents

Disclaimer

This publication is for informational purposes only and is not intended as medical advice. Medical advice should always be obtained from a qualified medical professional for any health conditions or symptoms associated with them.

Every possible effort has been made in preparing and researching this material. We make no warranties with respect to the accuracy, applicability of its contents or any omissions.

See your healthcare professional before starting any diet, health or exercise program!

Introduction

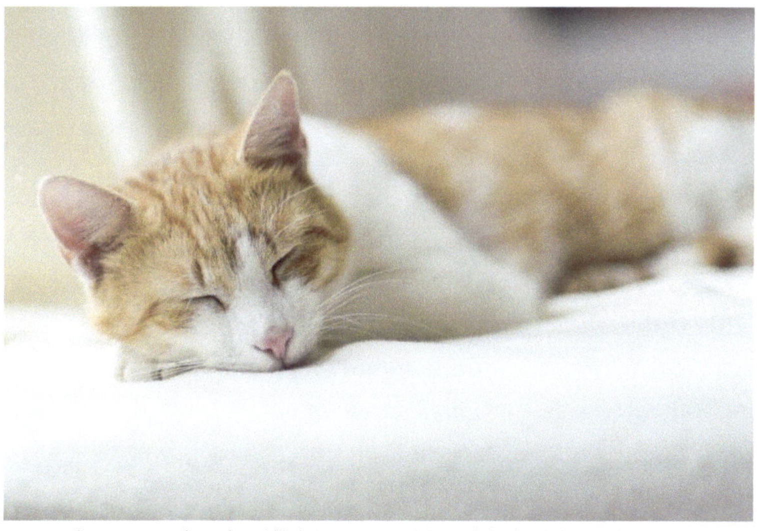

Clean eating was (and still is) a good health habit to have, but it and exercising will only take you so far in your journey for a healthy lifestyle. Why? Because if you are not getting the correct amount of quality sleep, your body does not have adequate time to rebuild itself overnight. Enter the newest health trend – Sleeping Clean. But what exactly does that mean? How do you sleep clean?

It isn't about washing your bedding more frequently or taking a shower before going to bed, although showering or taking a hot bath are both known to help you sleep better; it is much more than that. It focuses on preparing your body and environment so that both promote the highest quality and quantity of sleep.

Clean sleep evolution

Sleep studies have been going on for a number of years, however, the results were usually limited to being published in medical publications.

However that all changed when wellness aficionado and actress Gwyneth Paltrow and her GOOP Team discuss the value of sleep from a beauty and health perspective in their book ***Clean Beauty*** *(available from Amazon in either Kindle or hardcover formats at:* http://amzn.to/2iQ5o7L*)*.

In an article for Daily Mail.com Paltrow writes this about sleep *"You might think it's just a midlife thing, but if you find yourself feeling irritable, anxious, or depressed, if you get easily frustrated, forgetful, or struggle to cope with stress like you used to, it could be because you're not getting enough good-quality sleep. The lifestyle I lead is based not just on clean eating, but also on clean sleeping: at least seven or eight hours of good, quality sleep—and ideally even ten."* Since then, several articles have been published in various mainstream media exalting the health benefits of getting enough quality sleep, and health issues that can result from poor or not enough sleep.

Because sleep affects every aspect of the body, it should be prioritized just like any other health goal, including diet and exercise. Not getting enough quality or quantity of sleep can lead to a host of health issues, like:

- slowed metabolism
- hormone imbalance
- weight gain
- bad moods
- impaired memory, and brain fog
- inflammation and reduced immunity which can increase your risk of chronic disease
- increased aging
- reduced driving reaction time
- and many more

Because sleep is so important, you need to build time for it into your day, just like diet and exercise. It is **the** most important thing you can do for your overall physical and mental health.

The good news is that getting a good night's rest is totally doable, no matter how busy you are. Let's get started …

Curb Sleep Impairing Habits

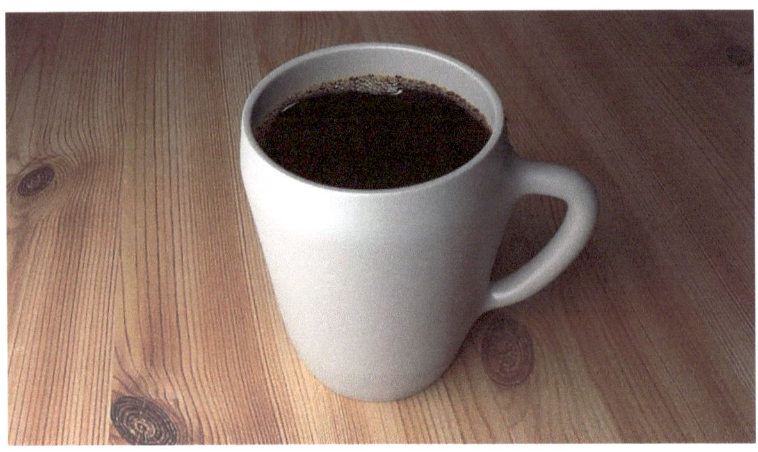

How do you know if you are getting enough sleep or not? One way to tell is if you go to sleep the minute your head hits your pillow. If you are getting enough sleep, then it should take 10 to 15 minutes to fall asleep. However, if you are still staring at the ceiling after 30 minutes or more, one or more of these nighttime habits may be the culprit.

Caffeine

Many of us use caffeine in our coffee in the morning as a pick-me-up, so why in the world would anyone drink it late in the day? It will have the same effect and could be the reason you are having trouble falling asleep.

However you may be eating foods late in the day that unknowingly contain caffeine and that could be impacting your sleep. Be sure to read the ingredients and nutritional label.

If your body is sensitive to caffeine, then you should quit drinking it early in the afternoon. For some people, the "kick" can last up to 10 hours.

Alcohol

A glass or wine or a nightcap may help you fall asleep, but it can prevent you from getting the quality REM sleep later on during the night. If you don't know, it is the REM phase that is the best as far as brain and body restoration. It's O.K. to have one 4-ounce glass of wine with dinner, but make sure it is at least three hours before your bedtime.

Blue light screens

Scientists have found that the blue light emitted by electronics, like tablets, laptops and phones – the devices commonly used right before bed or even after in bed – suppress melatonin production.

Melatonin is a natural occurring hormone that controls your bio-rhythms. As the light of day decreases, the body naturally increases melatonin to help you get sleepy and eventually fall to sleep. But if you are using a blue screen device, your body is not sensing the decrease of daylight.

If you're feel you have to use a blue screen device late in the day, try changing the screen to a more reddish color. Not only will it be easier on your eyes, but won't interfere with the production of melatonin.

Watching TV

Most TVs are nothing more than big blue screen devices, the same logic pertains to them as far as melatonin. Plus depending on what you watch, it could get your mind racing making it harder for your brain to settle down.

Exercising

Multiple studies have shown that working out can help you sleep better … but only if you do it correctly.

In one study, the participants who did at least 2.5 hours of moderate-to-vigorous activity per week resulted in a 65% improvement in sleep quality. And they reported feeling more alert the next day.

However, the time of day the exercising took place can also impact on sleep. Generally speaking, you shouldn't exercise any later than three hours before your bedtime. But because everyone is different, experiment with your exercise times to see what works best for you.

Eating spicy foods

Indigestion is never a good thing to help you fall asleep. So that late night pizza may have sounded like a good idea at the time, except now you can't go to sleep.

Avoid eating anything – especially spicy foods – that might upset your stomach close to bedtime. Again, three hours seems like the best time to stop eating. Experts agree that a light snack of maybe cereal and fruit, or nut butter or hummus on crackers should be fine, if you are concerned that hunger will keep you awake.

Room Temperature

Some people think it is easier to fall asleep in a warm room, because it makes you sleepy. However, at room temperature between 60 to 67 degrees Fahrenheit is the optimal temperature to help you fall sleep faster.

Working late

There are a couple of things working against you when working late. One, is most likely you are working on a device with a blue screen and we know how that impacts sleep. Two, you are not giving your brain the time it needs to wind down. You can't go from working to sleeping that fast.

Instead, wind down with something you enjoy that is relaxing to you, like some soft music or reading a book (but not on a bluescreen device!). Of course if you don't get a good night's sleep, you won't be able to perform at your best the next day. So did working late really accomplish anything as far as overall performance? Probably not.

If you are having trouble getting enough hours of sleep or good quality sleep, try one or more of these suggestions and see if your sleep improves.

Foods to Eat and Avoid to Sleep Better

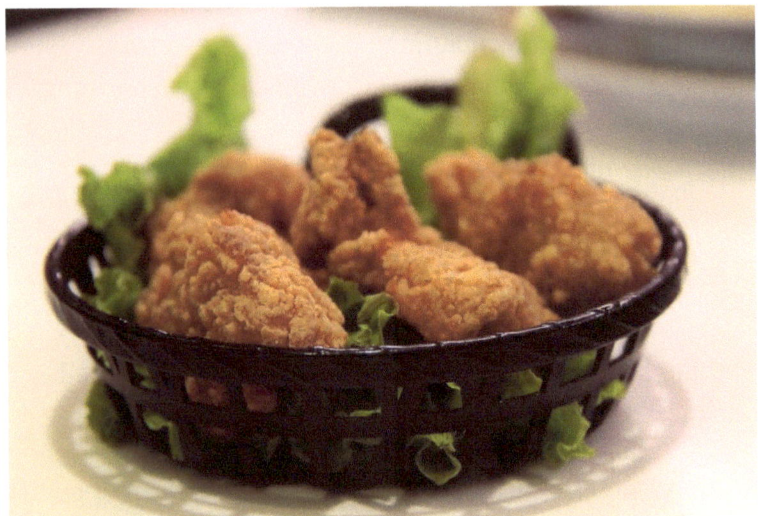

In the last chapter, we talked about how eating spicy foods right before bedtime can affect your sleep. In this chapter, we explore the topic of food further and its effect on sleep in more detail. Eating and sleeping are two of the basic human needs that go hand-in-hand in many ways. So, it's no surprise that what you eat before going to bed can affect the quality of your sleep – both good and bad.

So whether you sleep great or not can come down having eaten any of the best or worst foods, respectively before nodding off.

The best foods for sleeping well include:

- Melatonin-rich foods
- Warm drinks
- High Glycemic carbs
- High-Casein Dairy

Melatonin-rich foods

You don't have to supplement your diet with a melatonin tablet to boost your levels of the sleep-inducing hormone. Drinking a glass of tart cherry juice or eating a handful of walnuts every day can add about an hour and a half to your sleep time each night.

Warm Drinks

Drinking a warm glass of milk before going to bed has always been good advice for falling asleep. But do you know why it works? Dairy products are rich in tryptophan, calcium and vitamin D — all of which have been linked to improved sleep — but it works even better when it is warmed up first. Drinking a warm glass of milk raises your core temperature. In response, your body tries to get rid of the elevated heat by dilating blood vessels. This is the same exact process that occurs naturally that helps you fall asleep; warm milk just accelerates the process. Hot caffeine-free teas will also work in the same way.

High-Glycemic Carbs

Researchers believe foods with a high glycemic value like white rice, increase insulin levels in the body, which in turn stimulate the release of more tryptophan and melatonin, both hormones that help you fall asleep. Because turkey is also high in tryptophan, it works well too, as will bananas and granola because of their high GI level.

High-Casein Dairy

As evidenced by turkey, eating protein boosts the sleep-inducing hormone tryptophan. But there is something even better - casein protein.

By eating a slow-digesting form of that protein, like the kind found in cottage cheese or Greek yogurt, you increase your bodies' ability to recover from a workout and build muscle all night while you are stacking up the zzzzs.

Here are some foods to avoid as they can either prevent you from falling asleep or interrupt your sleep during the night:

- Alcohol
- Fried foods
- Caffeine
- Spicy foods

Alcohol

Who doesn't like a drink to help relax you so you can fall asleep, but it is also known to interrupt your sleep during the night, thus preventing you from getting your full REM sleep – the best quality sleep. Having a nightcap before going to bed can induce changes in brain waves similar to what happens with electric shock treatments. To keep that nightly toddy from interfering with your sleep, have it at least an hour before going to bed.

Fried Foods

Your night-time meal should be something light. Eating a heavy meal shortly before going to bed is a recipe for either acid reflux, which prevents you from sleeping, or can increase the production of the hormone dopamine which increases wakefulness. Your big heavy meal of the day should be at lunchtime, so your body has time to process it before the end of the day.

Caffeine

We know caffeine is all about staying awake. But in some people that are extra sensitive to the effects of caffeine, they should have their last coffee call well ahead of bedtime. Not only is coffee the culprit, but some teas and dark chocolate can produce the waking effect too.

Spicy Foods

Avoid eating any spicy foods within three hours of bedtime. Not doing so invites a bout with indigestion and acid reflux – both sleep interrupters. Have that bowl of chili for lunch instead and then something light for dinner.

Avoid This One Sleep-Sabotaging Habit

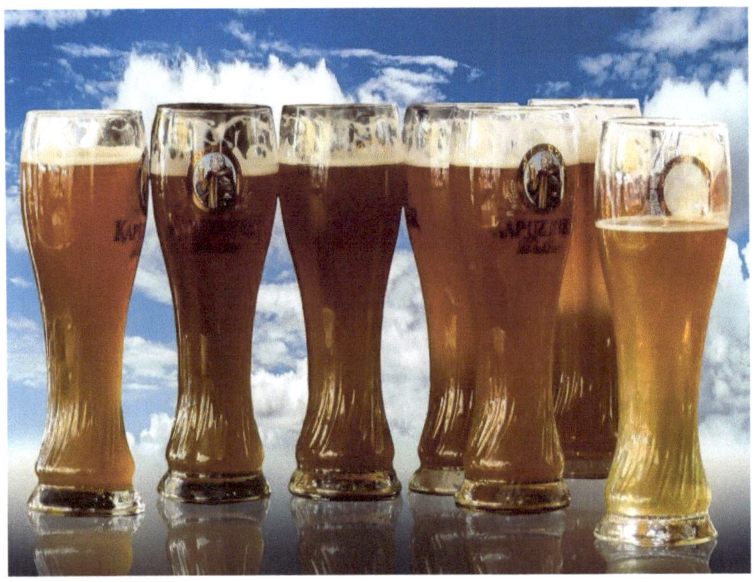

We briefly touched on the subject of alcohol in the last chapter; because it is so common for people to do, we wanted to delve deeper into the subject and why it is bad for sleep.

It can be one of those good-idea-at-the-time type of relaxers. I'll just have a glass of wine or two to unwind from the day and help me fall asleep. And it can make you drowsy in the beginning and help you get to sleep, but the downside is it can also erode your sleep quality later on in the night.

Why Alcohol

As a sedative, alcohol can make us feel a little buzzed, relaxed and helps us nod off quicker. However, just because a drink or two can make you fall asleep faster, it doesn't mean you'll get the quality, restorative sleep that makes us feel so rested the next day.

While asleep, our brain controls many of the body's important physiological functions, such as muscle growth, tissue repair and memory consolidation – a "cleaning" of the brain if you will. But having alcohol in your system can thwart some of these processes. But even more than that, alcohol does these other four things to interrupt your good quality sleep:

1. You have to get up to use the bathroom.
Our body uses a series of anti-diuretic hormones to keep enough water in our system so our blood pressure stays regulated. Alcohol can block the release of these hormones thus making you get up during the night to use the bathroom.

2. You sweat profusely.
Because only one or two drinks can increase the body temperature, the body responds by dilating the blood vessels in an attempt to regulate body temperature. This vasodilator effect results in sweating, making it uncomfortable for you to sleep. It is these night sweats that can make you toss and turn and rob of the valuable REM sleep.

3. Your blood sugar drops.
Depending on the type of drink, it could have a substantial amount of sugar in it. When drinking before going to bed, your body will release insulin in an attempt to process the sugar. But it may release too much, thus sending your blood sugar level down – and waking you up wanting that during-the-night carb snack.

4. Your REM sleep suffers.
Even moderate doses of alcohol can reduce the amount of time spent in REM sleep the type of good quality sleep Why is important?

Sleep is divided into two kinds: REM and non-REM. Scientists believe REM sleep is important for learning, memory consolidation and brain development, and is the reason why infants spend get more REM sleep than adults do. In one study, participants were taught a new skill.

Those that had sufficient REM sleep could recall what they learned, but those deprived of REM sleep could not.

The Takeaway

A good night's sleep is essential to recharge both your brain and body. But how much is required? In general at least seven hours of sleep per night ensuring all the hours are as restful as possible; as we will see later on in the book, nine hours are even better.

Because alcohol can negatively affect your sleep, try to enjoy it as far from bedtime as possible. However if you must have a drink before retiring, limit it to one drink (5-ounce serving of wine, 12-ounce beer or one mixed drink).

10 Tips to Improve Your Sleep

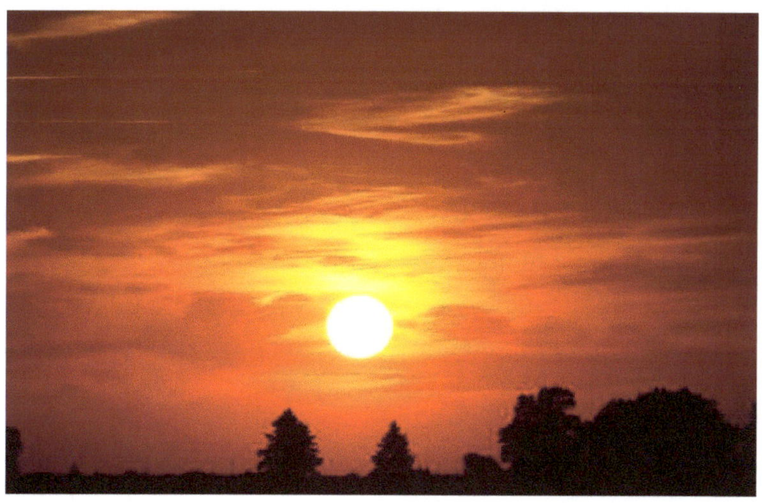

We all know how important a good night's sleep is to our overall health and workout recovery. However, aches and pains, stress, eating too late and a restless mind can sometimes keep us from getting the amount or quality of sleep we need. In fact, three out of five people don't get enough sleep. It is sleep deprivation that makes the day drag by at a snail's pace, reduces productivity, affects memory and even impairs driving. Law enforcement rates impairment from a lack of sleep right up there with other types of impairment including alcohol and drugs.

However, if you are not getting enough sleep, use these tips from experts to help you wake up refreshed and ready to meet the day head-on.

1. Take a warm bath. There is nothing more relaxing before bedtime than taking a warm bath scented with the essential oil lavender or having a scented candle lit in the bathroom.

2. Avoid confrontational TV programs prior to bedtime.
Watching these programs can get your mind racing instead of relaxing it making it harder, if not impossible, to fall asleep. Instead read a book while listening to soft music. It will put your body into a better pre-sleep state.

3. Stop drinking fluids three hours before bed. While we all know the value of staying hydrated during the day, it is best to stop drinking fluids three hours before retiring for the evening. This way you'll avoid the nightly ritual of having to go to the bathroom during the middle of the night, thus getting more or the beneficial REM sleep.

4. Turn off your computer and bright lights. Bio-rhythms to a certain extent are driven by the amount of daylight-colored light coming into our eyes. However blue screen devices, like tablets, laptops and smartphones emit a light similar in wavelength to daylight, thus preventing our body from secreting the hormone melatonin - the stuff that help us get sleepy and fall asleep. Instead, try dimming the lights and reading a hardcover book instead of an e-reader to relax.

5. Sleep on a firmer mattress. Supporting your cervical and lumbar spine by sleeping on a stiff mattress is one key to a more restful night. Not only will you wake up more refreshed, but also avoid waking up with a stiff neck and other pains caused by too soft of a bed.

6. Avoid beta blockers. Some medications contain beta-blockers which are known to cause insomnia in some people. If you take medication with beta-blockers, these could be the reason you are not sleeping soundly. Ask your doctor is there is something without beta-blockers you can take instead, or if not, if the dosage can be reduced.

7. Get plenty of real sunlight during waking hours. As noted before, light mimicking sunlight at bedtime prevents you from falling asleep. That is why is it wise to avoid blue screen devices right before falling asleep.

However getting real sunlight during the day, and avoiding that wavelength of light before bedtime, can help set your circadian clock, thus helping your body better determine when it time to start winding down. Couple this with a relaxing scented warm bath with soft music and you have a recipe for a restful night's sleep.

8. Avoid alcohol and caffeine before bedtime. Both of these liquids disrupt the transition our body needs to make to get into the REM-type of sleep. Plus they make us get up and go to the bathroom during the night further disrupting our REM sleep. This leads to sleep deprivation and we already know the problems that can cause.

9. Keep the bedroom cooler. Sometimes the sleep-disrupting culprit can be too hot of a bedroom temperature. Optimally an environment that is 60 to 65 degrees is the best for quality sleep. Any warmer and it can not only make it harder to fall asleep but disrupt your sleep during the night.

10. Practice slow breathing. This part of meditation can be a real boost in relaxing the body before bedtime. People have even fallen asleep during meditation sessions, so we know it works. Why not incorporate slow breathing into your bedtime routine and see if it helps you sleep better. You have nothing to lose and everything to gain.

Still feeling sleep deprived?

If none of these tips seem to be working for you, maybe something else is at play. See your healthcare professional to determine if you could be suffering from something else that could be causing interruption of your sleep, such as depression, anxiety, anemia or another condition called sleep apnea.

To improve recovery after a workout or be at your best performance-wise, don't overlook the tips in this chapter and your sleep patterns. Try to establish a daily pattern of sleep/awake so your body gets used to a routine.

Soon you'll be getting the restful quality and quantity of sleep that you need to wake up refreshed and ready to meet the day!

6 Ways to Slog Through the Day After a Bad Night's Sleep

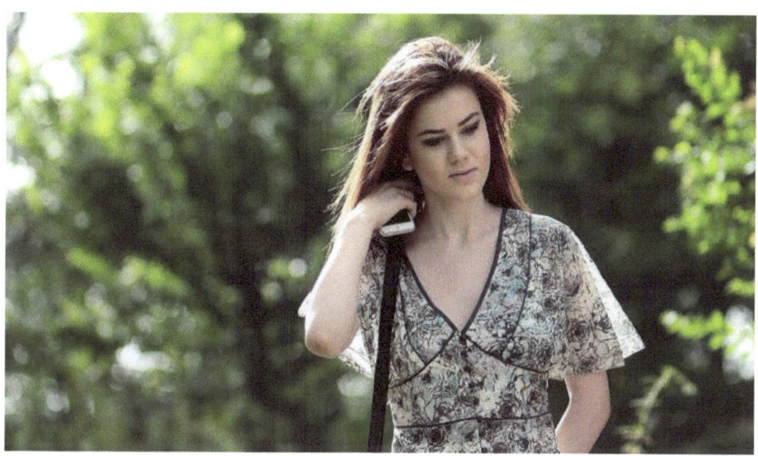

It is hard to get up and go to work or even get through the day, after having a bad night of sleep. Here are six things you can do to get you through it and get your body back on track:

1. Don't drink too much coffee late in the day. It is natural that you might want to grab a cup of coffee (or two or three) go help perk you up. However depending on how the caffeine affects you, stop drinking (or eating) anything with caffeine after lunch; that includes coffee, tea, energy drinks and chocolate. You want to make sure its effects are out of your system well before it is time to go to bed.

2. Eat breakfast. After fasting all night, you will want to "break your fast". Have something substantial that includes protein and carbs. Hot cereal with fruit and nuts or scrambled eggs and toast are good examples. Try to keep your blood sugar level on an even keel by eating regular meals and healthy snacks in between. Be sure to stay hydrated throughout the day.

3. Get outside at lunchtime. Going for a walk outside is refreshing and a great stimulate for the mind. Just leave enough time to stay outside and eat your healthy brown bag lunch you brought from home. Because sleep deprivation can cause anxiety and stress, getting some exercise will reduce it and its effects, thus helping you better get through the afternoon.

4. Don't crash on the couch. As tempting as it might be after you get home from work, don't do it. Keep moving until it is bedtime. This way it is easier to get your body back on its circadian rhythm schedule.

5. Eat a light supper, and a light snack 30 to 60 minutes before going to bed, if you are hungry. But you don't want to eat a heavy meal and have your digestive system work all night trying to process it. And a big meal could induce acid reflux which could prevent you from getting a good night's sleep again – making it two nights in a row.

6. Prep for tomorrow. I know you are tired and just want to go to bed. But spending a few minutes now getting everything ready for tomorrow will take the pressure off of you in the morning. Maybe you could even sleep in a little later than normal knowing you have everything ready to go for the day.

Don't Make This Number 1 Sleep Mistake!

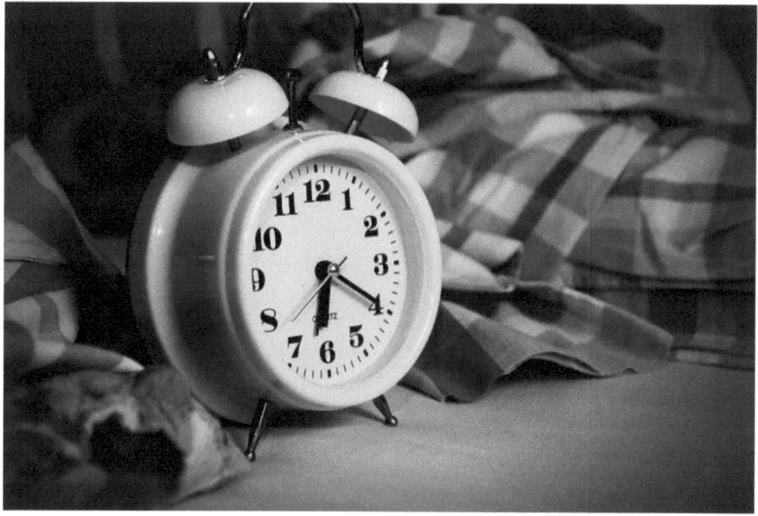

With sleep, quality is just as important as quantity. At night when we are sleeping, our brain is hard at working doing some "housekeeping" of the body. But did you know that sleep also keeps us healthy. Maintaining a healthy weight, improving our physical fitness and recharging our "battery" are only a few of the things that sleep does for us. Don't get enough or of good enough quality, and our body (and mind) suffer.

But sleeping does something else: it sets our internal clock and keeps us on an even circadian schedule. Without that schedule, many people function as sleep-deprived … even though they may be getting the required hours of sleep. When your life and circadian rhythm line up with each other, your body gets the right cues in many things – getting up and going to bed are just two of them. Without a consistent, schedule your body struggles to give you the right cues when you need them.

While going to bed at the same time each night is important, it is more important to get up at a consistent time. Timing is everything. Try to get up when the first rays of sun start to shine. By doing so, sunlight travels through the openings in your eyes, follows along the optic nerve to a part of the brain called the suprachiasmatic nucleus. It is this part of the brain that controls the body's sleep/wake cycle. Setting your wake time, helps your body establish your time to go to sleep.

Also there isn't such a thing as making up for lost sleep or banking sleep if you know you are going to have a late night. Sleep is only in the present, you can't do anything about lost sleep last night or sleep you are going to lose tomorrow night. However, short naps on the day after a short night's sleep can help add to your total number of hours of sleep for that day.

Some people work swing or night shifts which can be hard to get the body used to. But something even harder is rotating shifts. Your body no sooner gets used to one sleep/wake cycle and it is time to change to another. This is one reason why shift work is so hard on the body. It messes up the body's circadian rhythm.

Why Is 9 the Magic Number?

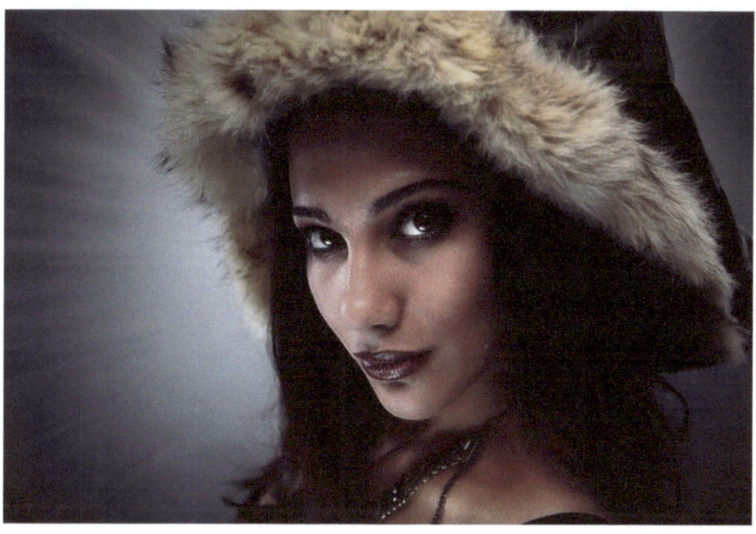

The amount and quality of sleep not only has a lot to do with your health, but also appearance. Gracefully aging, enjoying glowing skin and lush hair has to do with as much getting nine hours of good sleep every single night as it does anything else.

Why does sleep affects one's appearance? Because when we are sleeping is when the body repairs and detoxifies itself - the processes that allows you to look your best the next day.

But for women approaching menopause, their sleep can get interrupted by changes to their hormone levels. Early signs can range from night sweats to alertness during the middle of the night. This can leave one sleep-deprived the next day and stumbling through life.

However getting the right amount of sleep is crucial in helping maintain the correct level of hormones, so the amount one gets has a direct effect on one's youthful appearance.

When your sleep is poor in quality and quantity, your hormone output is inevitably affected; one of the most obvious signs is the dreaded middle-age spread.

Tiredness is seen by the body as a stressor; stress stimulates the production of the hormones cortisol and insulin, which triggers your body to store fat. But stress also works against you in another way; it reduces glucagon, the hormone that instructs your body to burn fat. So that lack of sleep gives you a double whammy; not only does it tell your body not to burn fat, it also tells it to store fat. This is why getting the proper amount and type of sleep is so important, because lack of sleep disrupts our metabolism and hormonal balance leading to weight gain.

Sleep deprivation can also increase the production of thyroxine, which over time can affect the functioning of your thyroid which also leads to weight gain and fatigue.

… and it isn't over yet. Sleep deprivation can cause a drop in the levels of appetite suppressant leptin, leaving you feeling hungry and more likely to overeat. It also causes the levels of the appetite-stimulating hormone ghrelin to rise, increasing your hunger and appetite, particularly for carbohydrates.

So just a lack of sleep over time can cause all these things to work against you as far as trying to maintain a healthy appearance as far as weight. Just another reason why getting nine hours of restful sleep per night is so important.

4 Cleaver Ways to Sleep Clean

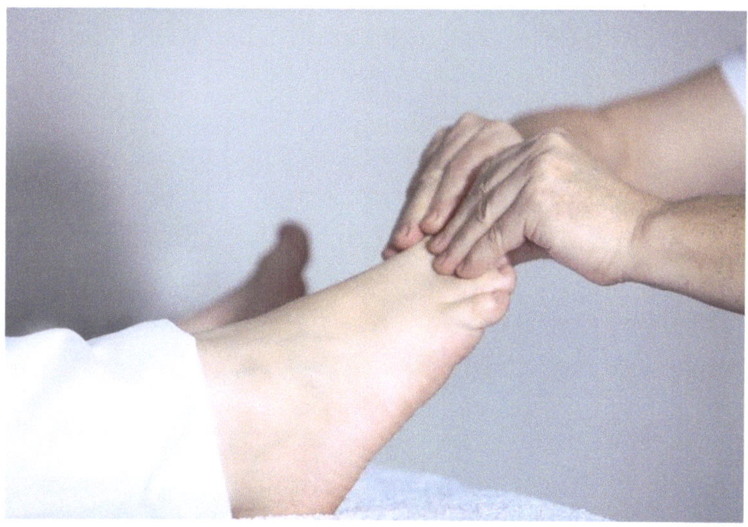

A form of meditation called yoga nidra, meaning "psychic sleep" is a form of meditation you can do at home that is believed to give you the benefits of sleep while you're awake. While you can find many guided sessions of how to do it online, you can try this by yourself:

Lie down, close your eyes and simply try to focus (in relatively quick succession) on individual parts of the body, as you cast your attention in a circular motion from one hand — each finger, one by one — to your palm, wrist, forearm, elbow, upper arm, shoulder, neck, face, etc., and down the other arm across to the torso, down one leg and up the other.

With practice, you can even include internal organs in the circuit. Meditating like this takes your body and brain to a point that is very close to sleep, with all its restorative benefits, and the effect can be deeply relaxing.

Ban during-the-night snacks

Running to the refrigerator for a mid-night snack can disrupt sleep because of the digestive process required to break down the snack you just had. Plus depending on what you ate, acid reflux could result further eroding the sleep you need.

Your digestive system needs a break at night; that is why it is called a "fast". For your body to really to cleanse itself overnight, keep to a regular 12-hour fasting schedule — so if you finish last food at 8.30pm, you shouldn't "break fast" until breakfast after 8.30am the next day.

Your body won't slip into deep detox mode until about eight hours after your last meal and then it needs about four more hours of undisturbed sleep to do its job properly.

Rub your head's trigger points

On the back of your head are "trigger points" that when massaged correctly can have therapeutic effects.

Working the trigger points can stimulate circulation, disperse accumulated toxins and speed the flow of oxygenated blood throughout the body. Not only can this help you think more clearly, it can also relieve tension headaches, sinus issues and helps reduce fatigue and insomnia.

To use this therapy, place your hands on the back of your head and move four to five finger-widths from the back of your ear to your hairline at the base of the skull. Use your left hand for the left side (and vice versa).

Massage these trigger points just before going to bed by applying gentle pressure with each thumb. When you've located the correct spot, you will feel an indentation and tender spot when you have hit the point.

To release each point of tension, move your thumb in a circular motion with gentle applied pressure for 10 seconds. Be sure to do the other side also.

Massage your feet

Your feet are a long way from your head, but because they are connected via your spinal column, massaging each of them with a super-rich thick cream for three minutes each can relieve mental tension built up from the day.

Just work the cream in gently (or have your significant other do it for you) and feel the tension flow out of your mind. Now you are prepared for truly restful sleep.

Buy a copper pillow

Copper has been known for a number of years to relieve certain aches and pains, but now scientists are finding out its value as a method to reduce the formation or wrinkles. By using a metal-infused pillow that uses fine strands of copper oxide in the material, they believe it helps boost elastin and collagen in the skin, along with having anti-microbial properties that fight bacteria and could help tame the dark spots and acne that can re-appear around middle age.

They think when your face is in contact with the pillowcase, copper ions are transferred into the upper layers of your skin, where they help support cell renewal.

Some pillows use a silver ion technology that also helps reduce harmful bacteria found on the face. Those pillows are usually made from cotton and infused with fine silver strands.

Final Thoughts

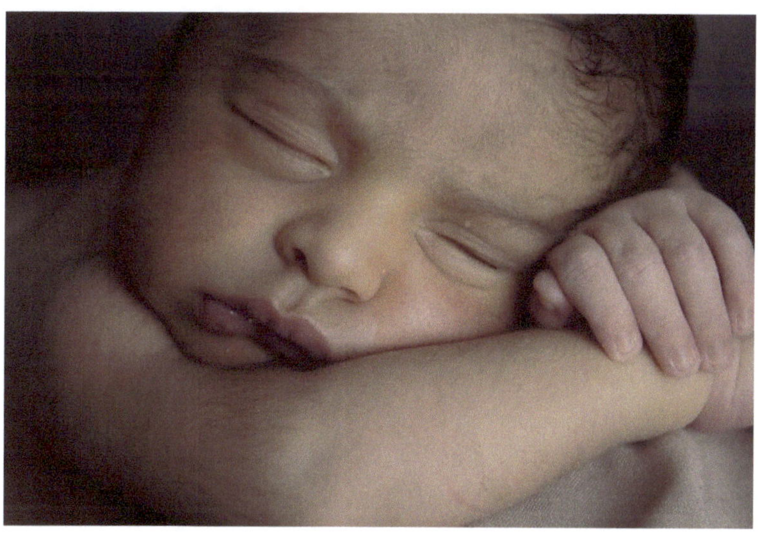

There are dozens of different types of sleep problems. Some of them are medical and some habitual, meaning habits created the problem. If you're dealing with a chronic sleep problem, it may be time to face the facts and get help. Let's take a look at the five most common reasons people don't get help for their sleep problems. Maybe you'll recognize yourself or someone you know in these scenarios.

1. They're Unaware They Have Sleep Problems but They Are Always Tired

Sleep apnea is a common sleep problem. It's a condition where you stop breathing during the night. You might stop for a few seconds or up to a full minute. And it can happen occasionally or several hundred times a night. The unusual thing about sleep apnea is that most people don't know that they have it. They're just tired all the time.

Most people with sleep apnea don't wake up when they stop breathing. But they are roused from deep and restful sleep to a lighter stage of sleep, which impacts their quality of sleep.

2. They Think They Can Handle It Themselves

There are some misunderstandings about many common sleep problems. For example, did you know that if you wake too early in the morning and cannot go back to sleep, that's insomnia? Or if you wake several times during the night that is also considered insomnia?

Most people who deal with this type of sleep problem don't actually think it's a problem. They assume that it's just part of life and they have to deal with it. They might take sleep aids to help get them through the night. Instead, going to the doctor to talk about insomnia treatments can help you get back to a consistently good night of sleep.

3. They Think It Will Pass

Most people deal with the occasional short-term bout of insomnia. It lasts for a few days and coincides with life's stress, illness, or a transition. However, if insomnia lasts for more than a few weeks, it's important to get help.

4. They Simply Adapt

Seniors are known for their tendency to go to bed early and wake up early. It's not uncommon to hear about someone who falls asleep right after dinner and wakes up around three or four in the morning. This adaptation actually interrupts your body's natural desire to wake and sleep on a 24-hour clock set by the sunlight. It impacts the quality of your sleep.

A doctor can help you get your body clock back on an optimal schedule with light therapy, melatonin, and behavioral therapy.

5. They Smoke but Don't Want to Quit

Finally, many people know the cause of their sleep problems and they're unwilling to change. For example, someone who smokes will often struggle with sleep apnea and restless sleeping. However, they're unwilling to quit smoking so they don't go to a doctor for their sleep problems.

Getting enough quality sleep every night is so important in many aspects of our life that if you are having problems sleeping well on a consistent basis, see your healthcare professional and get some help. They can identify the problem and suggest treatment to help you get a better night's sleep.

Other Relevant Books by This Author

If you would like to read more relevant books about this topic, here is a list of the CreateSpace links, titles and descriptions from this author:

https://www.amazon.com/Health-Wellness-Planning-Reports-Healthiest/dp/1541119185

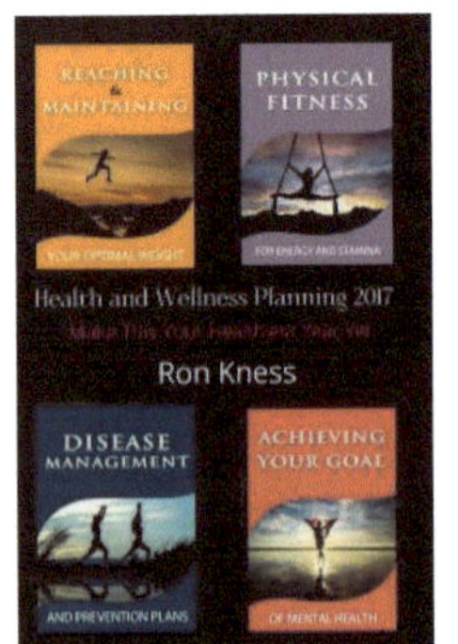

Health and Wellness Planning: 4 Reports to Help Make This Your Healthiest Year Yet

Your doctor is a valuable resource when it comes to your health and fitness concerns. However, many people don't know how to talk to their doctors.

After some visits, you might even leave the doctor's office with more questions than answers. Maybe you feel that you don't have a chance during your appointment to say what's really on your mind.

Talking to your doctor is very important before you begin any new fitness and exercise regimen, especially if you have been quite sedentary up until now. Here are some tips to help you prepare so you can leave your next appointment with the best answers possible.

- Bring up the topic of fitness and exercise yourself. If you wait for your doctor to mention it, the subject may not come up.

Some doctors are reluctant to bring up fitness and exercise because they don't want to hurt their patients' feelings.

- Prepare your questions ahead of time. Your doctor has budgeted only a certain amount of time to spend with you. You can make your appointment run more quickly and smoothly by writing down your questions ahead of time. When your appointment starts, let your doctor know that you have a list of questions. That will indicate to your doctor that you are seeking particular information and they will usually give you the opportunity to work your way through the list.

- Ask about what kinds of exercise you should be doing. Your doctor will know your medical history and will know if certain types of exercise would be unwise for you to try. They may be concerned about you getting injured. As well, if you have any medical conditions or are taking any medications, that might affect your ability to do certain exercises.

- Ask about your resting heart rate and what your target heart rate should be. Your doctor can explain these to you. Your doctor will be able to tell you what your target heart rate should be based on your age and medical condition. He or she can also show you how to easily calculate your heart rate.

- If you want to lose weight, this is a good opportunity to discuss a reasonable weight-loss goal with your doctor. He or she will be able to tell you what a realistic weight loss would be for your condition. They can also help you determine your ideal weight.

- Ask about diet and nutrition. Your doctor can tell you how many calories you should be eating each day to stay healthy and may recommend certain foods to improve and maintain your health.

- Take notes. While your doctor is speaking, take notes of their answers. With so much information being thrown at you, it will be impossible to remember all of it. You may also want to bring along a friend to ask any questions you didn't think of and to help remind you of important details after you leave.

Your doctor is an important partner in your health care. By taking this advice, you will be able to start a meaningful conversation with your doctor and gain helpful information.

In this book are four reports that after reading may help you better plan your next trip with your doctor in regard to health and fitness:
• Achieving Your Goal of Mental Health
• Disease Management and Prevention Plans
• Physical Fitness for Energy and Stamina
• Reaching and Maintaining Your Optimal Weight

These 4 reports will not only help you improve your health and wellness, but also serve to spur meaningful conversations with your doctor.

https://www.amazon.com/Productive-Mornings-Create-Ritual-Productivity/dp/1536982237

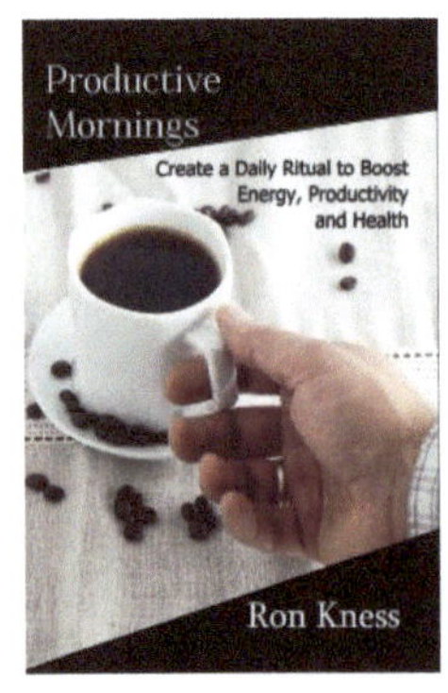

Productive Mornings: Create a Daily Ritual to Boost Energy, Productivity and Health

Most people admit to being less productive than they would like to be. Then there are those individuals that seem to be able to squeeze two or three days' worth of production out of a day's worth of time.

The result is definitely not a difference in willpower or effort. This is not a case where most unproductive people are lazy. On the contrary, many people work very hard at trying to be more productive, but continually fall short of their goals.

The difference between those two sets of people often times comes down to how they spend their mornings.
Do you wake up to an alarm clock at a specific time, or do you simply rise from your bed whenever you feel like it?

Do you follow the same process each morning, or do you just sort of "wing it", following no specific game plan? There is plenty of research to indicate that those people who wake up in the morning with a purpose and a plan enjoy wonderful benefits like better productivity, better health, greater happiness and other rewards.

In my book, we explore the benefits of a having a boost in energy and productivity, along with enjoying better health - three things all of us could use more of. We also lead you by the hand in creating your morning ritual.

https://www.amazon.com/Stress-Hormone-Cortisol-Chronic-Conditons/dp/153978598X

Ron Kness

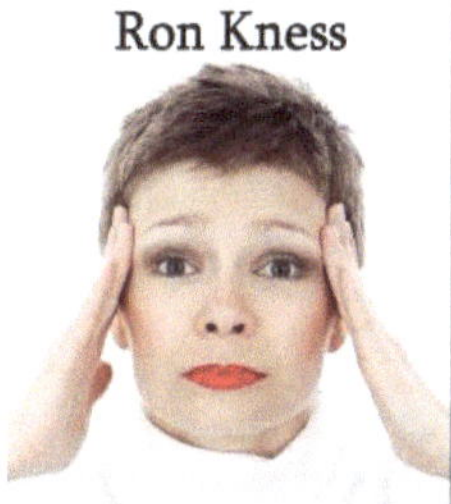

The Stress Hormone Cortisol

The Stress Hormone Cortisol: In Chronic Excess, It Can Be the Root Cause of Several Medical Conditions

A person who is under excessive stress is often described as someone who is always working "under the gun". This expression should be a fair indicator that too much exposure to stress is a big threat to a person's health and well-being.

Repeated studies expose the correlation between stress and ill-health, and why chronic stress is such an important health problem. Cortisol is a type of glucocorticoid hormone. Along with adrenaline, it is one of the main hormones responsible for stress responses.

The actions of cortisol in the human body are quite complex. As a primary stress hormone it not only acts directly on the body, but also acts indirectly by activating other hormones, each with a critical role to perform.

In a healthy person with a healthy cycle consisting of a stress incident followed by an adequate rest and recovery phase, cortisol has a major function of instigating homeostasis, or returning the body to normal after being exposed to stress.

This is enacted largely through the triggering of secondary hormones.

The recovery phase following an acute stress incident is critical for the prevention of developing chronic stress. Chronic stress develops when persistent stress causes stress hormones, including cortisol, to remain constantly elevated in the body. In this all too common situation, cortisol remains awash in the body at high levels for long periods of time.

Unfortunately in today's world, this is happening a lot. In my book, I look not only look at ways to reduce stress, but also some things you can do to better cope with stress.

About the Author

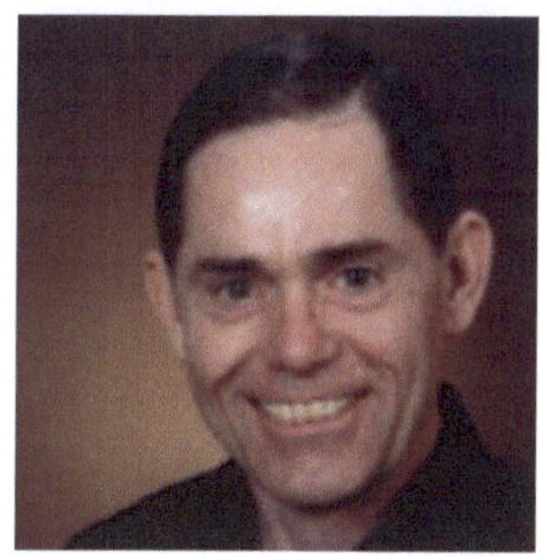

I grew up in Central Minnesota, where my parents owned and operated a fishing resort. Once out of high school I tried a couple of semesters of college, only to quit halfway through the Spring term; I decided at that time that college wasn't for me.

Then I decided to follow my father's previous occupation as an auto mechanic. I graduated from a two-year of vocational training course and worked as a mechanic for five years. While in vocational training, I decided to join the National Guard where I eventually ended up working full-time for 32 years.

So how does all of this relate to writing? In one of my leadership schools, the instructor, who was an English teacher at a juvenile detention center, presented writing to me in a whole new way - a way that started to develop my interest in working with words.

I eventually went back to college on the GI Bill while I was working and earned my Bachelor's degree in Business Administration. Taking a class or two per semester at night and on weekends took me seven years to complete my degree.

Fast forward about 40 years and I now have published over 100 books on Amazon for Kindle, CreateSpace and other publishing platforms.

Besides my own writing, I also ghostwrite ebooks, books, reports, articles, blogs and do Kindle conversions for clients on a variety of topics.

Today my wife and I are retired from our careers and live in Gold Canyon, AZ. I now write as a retirement business where you'll find me happily sitting in my office typing away on my laptop as I work on my next book or ghostwriting project . . . that is if we are not traveling on a cruise ship - our new-found mode of travel.

www.ingramcontent.com/pod-product-compliance
Lightning Source LLC
Chambersburg PA
CBHW040904260726
48664CB00025B/1443